Ways Microorganisms Stay, Enter The Body And Disease Prevention

Olatundun Solomon

olatundunsolomon@gmail.com

1. Drinking Dirty Water:
Dirty water can contain disease causing microorganisms(pathogens). When this dirty water is taking into the body through the mouth, it can cause infection. This can result to sickness.

Prevention is by drinking clean water.

2. Bathing With Dirty Water:

Dirty water can contain disease causing microorganisms(pathogens). Bathing with it can cause skin disease.

Prevention is by bathing with clean water.

3. Using Dirty Water To Wash Clothes:

Dirty water can contain disease causing microorganisms(pathogens). Using this dirty water to wash clothes can make infection of skin to occur after wearing the clothes. This can result to skin disease.

Prevention is by using clean water to wash clothes.

4. Using Dirty Water To Wash Plates, Spoons And Pot:

Dirty water can contain disease causing microorganisms(pathogens). Using it to wash plates, spoons and pot when the pot is used to prepare food and the spoons and plates are used to eat, it can cause transfer of the microorganisms to the body. This can result to disease in the body.

Prevention is by using clean water to wash plates, spoons and pot.

5. From The Cough Of An Infected Person:

From the cough of an infected person.

Somebody that is close by can be infected. This can result to disease.

The infected person can go to the hospital for treatment. The infected person can use handkerchief to cover mouth and nose when coughing to prevent the spread of infection.

6. From Dirty Hands:

Dirty hands can have disease causing microorganisms. When the hands are not washed and are used to eat it can result to disease in the body.

Prevention is washing hands with soap and water.

7.Untreated Open wounds:

When there is open wounds. Disease causing microorganisms in the air can stay on the open wounds. This can cause disease of the body.

Prevention is going to the hospital for treatment of open wounds.

8. Using Dirty Water To Wash The Face:

Dirty water can contain disease causing microorganisms(pathogens).

This can cause eye and skin disease.

Prevention is using clean water to wash the face.

9. Using Dirty Earbuds:

The dirty earbuds can contain disease causing microorganisms. This can cause ear disease.

Prevention is use clean earbuds.

10. Wearing Dirty Clothes:

Dirty clothes can contain disease causing

microorganisms. This can cause skin disease.

Prevention is wear clean clothes.

11. Wearing Dirty Shoes:

Dirty shoes can contain disease causing microorganisms. This can cause disease to occur to the feet.

Prevention is wear clean shoes.

12. Wearing Dirty Cap:

Dirty cap can contain disease causing microorganisms. Wearing such a cap can cause disease to occur to the head.

Prevention is wear clean cap.

13. Dirty Handkerchief:

Dirty handkerchief can contain disease causing microorganisms. When the dirty handkerchief is used on the body, it can make disease to occur.

Prevention is use clean handkerchief.

14. Dirty Bed:

Dirty bed can contain disease causing microorganisms (pathogens).

Sleeping on dirty bed can make disease to occur to the skin.

Prevention is sleep on clean bed.

15. Dirty Car:

Dirty car can contain disease causing microorganisms (pathogens).

Driving a dirty car can cause disease causing microorganisms to be in clothes. This can cause disease to occur to the skin.

Prevention is drive clean car.

16. Dirty Phone:

Dirty phone can have
disease causing
microorganisms
(pathogens) on it.

When dirty phone is
continually used, it can
cause skin disease.

Prevention is use clean
phone.

17. Dirty Pen:

Dirty pen can have disease causing microorganisms (pathogens) on it.

When dirty pen is continually used, it can cause skin disease.

Prevention is use clean pen.

18. Dirty Pencil:

Dirty pencil can have disease causing microorganisms (pathogens) on it.

When dirty pencil is continually used, it can cause skin disease.

Prevention is use clean pencil.

19. Dirt Wardrobe:

Dirty wardrobe can contain disease causing microorganisms (pathogens)

When dirty wardrobe is used. It can cause disease causing microorganisms to be in the clothes. This can cause skin disease.

Prevention is use clean wardrobe.

20. Dirty Food:

Dirty food can contain disease causing microorganisms(pathogens).

Eating dirty food can make disease to occur to the body.

Prevention is eat clean food.

21. Not Well Cooked Food:

When food is not well cooked it can have living disease causing microorganisms in it. When such food is eaten, it can cause disease to the body.

Prevention is cook food well.

22. Breathing Through Open Mouth:

Breathing through open mouth can cause disease causing microorganisms in the air by the force of the wind to enter into the body.

Prevention can be, breathe through the nose and move away from or take away dirts that are close by.

23. Breathing In Air In Affected Area:

Breathing in air in areas that are affected by disease causing microorganisms, can cause disease causing microorganisms to enter into the body through the

nose. This can cause
disease.

Prevention can be, move
away from or take away
dirts that are close by.

24. Wearing Dirty Socks:
Dirty socks can have
disease causing
microorganisms.

Wearing dirty socks can cause disease to occur to the legs.

Prevention is wear clean socks.

25. Wearing Dirty Hand gloves:

Dirty hand gloves can have disease causing microorganisms in them. Wearing dirty hand gloves can cause disease to occur to the skin of the hands.

Prevention is wear clean hand gloves.